Dreadlocks

Ultimate guide

Published by Smail Jarrou
First Edition

© Copyright 2021. All rights reserved

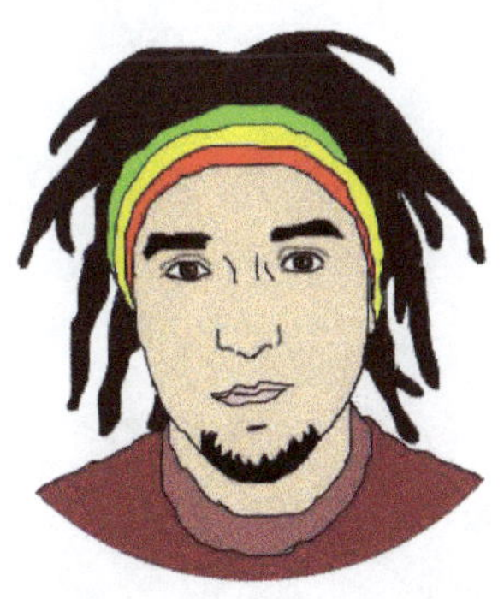

TABLE OF CONTENT

INTRODUCTION

DISCLAIMER

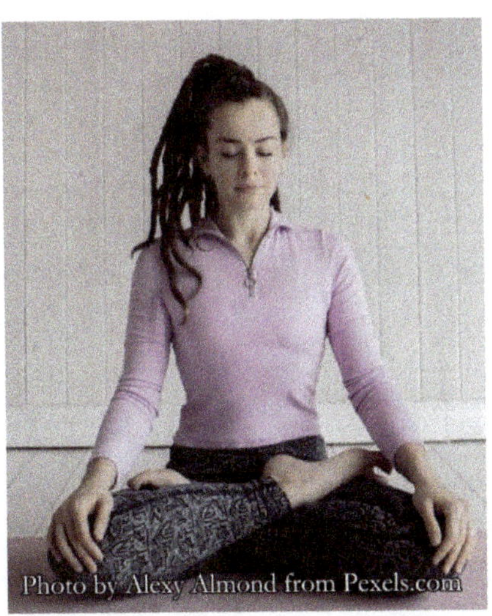

Photo by Alexy Almond from Pexels.com

The term "dreadlocks" is getting less and less popular with time, it is getting slowly replaced by other terms like "Locs" or "Locks". But you will find it all over the book for the simple reason that this book is basically made of blog articles that I wrote throughout the years when it was still ok to say dreadlocks or even just "dreads".
I still use the word "dreadlocks" in my blog posts though, for the sake of Search Engine Optimization and algorithms.

This book is about locs as a hairstyle and nothing else.
How to start your locs journey, how to take care of your hair... stuff like that. It is not intended to start a debate or to give answers about any cultural conflicts.

Dreadlocks suit everyone, anyone can have them regardless of their hair texture, with the difference that with some hair types you might need some extra work and extra time. But basically any hair that was left uncombed for a while will lock itself in a natural process.

<u>WELCOME</u>

If you are reading this book it's because you are interested in dreadlocks, you either have them, or you are planning to start a journey or maybe you are just curious. Welcome anyway, I will share with you the information that I gathered throughout my 10 years dreadlock Journey, about how to get them, how to maintain them.. and other related issues.

I decided to start writing because I have noticed in my humble experience that most people don't know much about dreadlocks, many are misinformed, and there are plenty of stereotypes. I felt that I needed to spread the truth about not something that I have tried but something that has become a part of me.

So here is my little contribution to the community: the story of a fellow dreadhead from Morocco - Africa.

Thank you for reading!

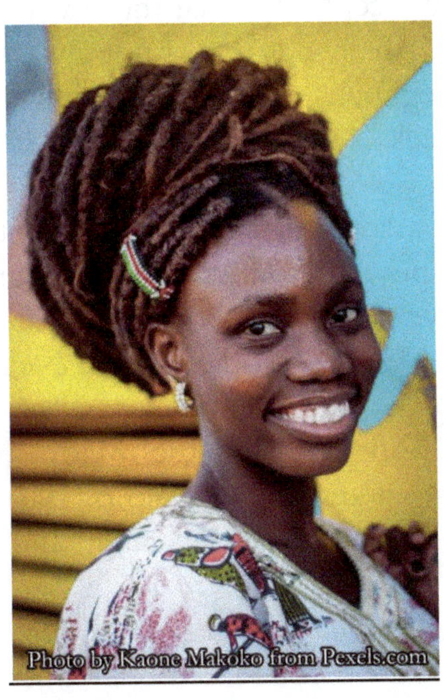
Photo by Kaone Makoko from Pexels.com

GENERAL INFO ABOUT DREADLOCKS

Dreadlocks, also called locks, locs, a ras, dreads, "rasta" or Jata (Hindi), are matted coils of hair. Dreadlocks are usually intentionally formed; because of the variety of different hair textures, various methods are used to encourage the formation of locks such as backcombing.

Additionally, leaving long hair to its own devices by not brushing or cutting the hair will encourage it to tangle together as it grows, leading to twisted, matted ropes of hair known as dreadlocks. The latter method is typically referred to as the neglect method.

A common misconception is that those who have dreadlocks do not wash their hair, but this is not always the case. Many dreadlock care regimens require the wearer to wash their hair up to twice a week (a normal amount for healthy, clean hair of any style).

Dreadlocks are associated most closely with the Rastafari movement, but people from many ethnic groups in history before them have worn dreadlocks, including many ancient Semitic and Indo-Aryan peoples of the Near East and Asia Minor, Sadhus of Nepal,

India and the Sufi Rafaees, the Māori people of New Zealand, the Maasai and the Oromo of East Africa, and the Sufi malangs and fakirs of Pakistan, and medieval Irish Warriors.

Etymology

The word is a compound word combining the words dread and locks that dates to the time of the invasion of native peoples in the West Indies. In the 1960s the intent may have been to evoke the dread aroused in beholders of the hair; "dread" also has a sense of "fear of the Lord" in the Rastafari Movement, which can be partially expressed as alienation from contemporary society.

History

The first known examples of dreadlocks date back to East Africa and some parts of North Africa.

Maasai men found in the regions of northern Tanzania and southern Kenya have been wearing dreadlocks for as long as they have survived.

There hasn't been official date of the "start" of Maasai dreadlocks, but it is a tradition that has been going on for thousands of years. Even today, Maasai men can be found easily donning their dreadlocks, with a tint of red color from the soil.

In ancient Egypt, examples of Egyptians wearing locked hairstyles and wigs have appeared on bas-reliefs, statuary and other artifacts. Mummified remains of ancient Egyptians with locks, as well as locked wigs, have also been recovered from archaeological sites.

The Hindu deity Shiva and his followers were described in the scriptures as wearing "jaTaa", meaning "twisted locks of hair", probably derived from the Dravidian word "Sadai", which means to twist or to wrap. The Greeks, the Pacific Ocean peoples, the Naga people and several ascetic groups within various major religions have at times worn their hair in locks, including the monks of the Ethiopian Orthodox Tewahedo Church, the Nazirites of Judaism, Qalandari Sufi's the Sadhus of Hinduism, and the Dervishes of Islam among others. The very earliest Christians also may have worn this hairstyle. Particularly noteworthy are descriptions of James the Just, first Bishop of Jerusalem, who wore them to his ankles.

Pre-Columbian Aztec priests were described in Aztec codices (including the Durán Codex, the Codex Tudela and the Codex Mendoza) as wearing their hair untouched, allowing it to grow long and matted.

In Senegal, the Baye Fall, followers of the Mouride movement, a sect of Islam indigenous to the country which was founded in 1887 by Shaykh Aamadu Bàmba Mbàkke, are famous for growing locks and wearing multi-colored gowns. Cheikh Ibra Fall, founder of the Baye Fall school of the Mouride Brotherhood, popularized the style by adding a mystic touch to it, it's important to note that warriors among fullani, wolof, serer and mandika were also known to have dreadlocks when old and cornrows when young for centuries.

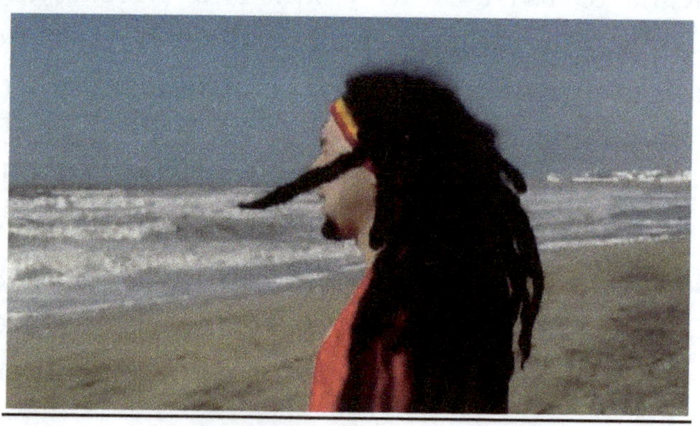

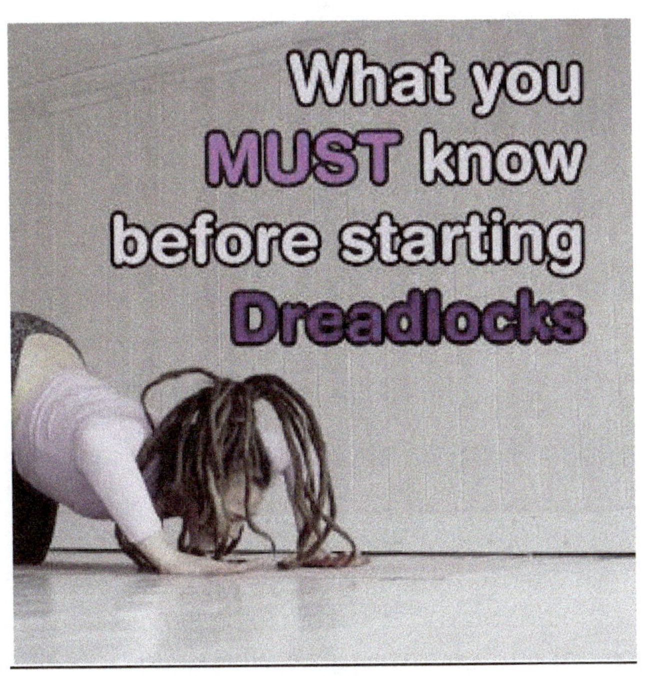

WHAT YOU NEED TO KNOW BEFORE STARTING YOUR LOCS JOURNEY

If you are considering starting your first dreadlocks journey then there are few things you need to be aware of.

Questions to ask yourself and to think deeply of before locking your hair

1- What does the word "dreadlocks" mean?

This simply means that you have to collect as many information as you can about dreads, from history, to cultures who had them as hairstyle, to dread's products you can use, to even the possible links between being a dreadhead and spirituality... etc

(You might come across some funny myths like that dreadlocks attract bugs or that your hair has to be dirty to lock...)

2- Why do you want to have dreadlocks?

There are so many reasons why people start their dreadlocks journey: trying something different, being or becoming a rasta, changing the look, trying to look like a celebrity, self-empowerment and growth... Knowing why YOU want to have them will help you a lot in the future, especially in choosing the dreadlocks method that suits you the most.

3- How patient are you?

Patience is crucial when it comes to dreadlocks, you will know later why you need a lot of it, if you're not patient enough then you should reconsider having locs, they are probably not for you.

General information about dreadlocks you must know

1- You will mostly not have the exact result you imagined

You probably wanted to have dreads like Bob Marley or any other celebrity that you admire, but you will probably not get the exact look you wanted length and size wise.

Your dreads will just do their thing they won't care about your wishes. So just be ready to accept whatever your hair ends up doing. Every dreadlocks journey is unique so be proud of yours.

2- You will have a messy hair for a while.

We are talking here about at least a year before your dreads mature, that's when you will need the "lots of patience" we talked about earlier. So be ready to deal with the mess on a daily basis, using bandanas or bonnets or any head accessories for your interlocking locs.

3- Washing your hair will be different.

There will be no brushing any more, which is going to be a challenge to get used to. You will also need to have a residue-free shampoo to help your hair locking. And finally every now and then you will have to do a deep cleaning, because no matter how good you wash your dreads they will still have build up inside that you have to do a cleaning and a "detoxing dreads", using Baking soda and apple cider vinegar for example.

4- Drying locs takes ages.

If washing your locked hair will be just a new different routine, drying it is another story. No matter what you do to your dreadlocks they will always take hours to dry after getting them wet, take that into consideration because it will change your daily plans.

Regardless of all these negative sides, having dreadlocks could be the best experience you might have in your life. They will boost your self confidence and make you feel special, because of course not everybody has the chance to have them. And above all my favorite part is that you will find a welcoming community in every social media platform that you can be a part of, which is very fun.

Dreadlocks might be a lot of work but the final result is totally worth it. Trust me.

HOW TO MAKE DREADLOCKS

So your hair is long enough now to start your dreadlocks journey?.. The next step is to choose the dreading method, depending on your hair type, and the patience degree you have.
Here are the different dreading methods that exist, with advantages and disadvantages of each one.
There will be a dedicated section for each method with more details.

1-NEGLECT METHOD:

How to do it: You don't do anything actually except washing your hair and not brushing it, you let it grow naturally. With time, after a year or so it will start to knot and to form dreads on itself, you might help it by separating the dreads while they are growing or by using rubber bands to define the sections, but the true neglect people don't do all this.

Advantages: easy to do, no tools or products needed, no assistance or help; It's the healthiest way to have healthy dreadlocks. No hair damages.

Disadvantages: Takes a lot of time, at least a year before the dreads start forming, or more if your hair is smooth and straight. dreads are not all of the same size, some are fat others are skinny, needs a lot of patience.

2-BACKCOMBING METHOD:

How to do the backcombing method: Section your hair in squares, big or small depending on the dreads size you want, start combing the hair backwards using a dread comb, you begin from the root of the hair to the tip of it; You may use rubber bands to secure your dreads and take them off later.

Advantages: you control the size of your dreads. they mature faster than other methods. it works on all kinds of hair especially straight Caucasian hair. It's almost an all natural method.

Disadvantages: Takes few hours to make. Needs someone to help you with. The process hurts sometimes. you may lose some hair in the process.

3-TWIST AND RIP METHOD:

How to do it: Section your hair in squares (depending on the size you want for your dreads). Split the sectioned part in two, hold each part in one hand, then twist clockwise, change the hands and spread the sectioned part till it gets tight by the root, repeat till you reach the end of hair. you might do some palm rolling afterwards.

Advantages: You control the size of your dreads. it's almost an all natural method (unless you use wax). your dreads look like real mature dreads the same day.

Disadvantages: doesn't work well for straight smooth hair. you may lose a little bit of hair in the process. may take time doing it and the making hurts a little bit as well.

4-DREAD PERMING METHOD:

How to do the perming method: Go to a salon that does it, and pay them to do it.

Advantages: after going out of the salon you will have dreadlocks instantly.

Disadvantages: It's a chemical process. Must be done by professionals. It will mostly damage your hair.

5-WOOL METHOD:

How to do the Wool dread method: Take a wool piece of clothing (sweater, hat or gloves) put it on your hair and rub it in circles for few minutes till you feel knots starting to form. You may rip it apart later to separately form your dreads.
Advantages: All natural method, no help needed, no tools (except wool hat).
Disadvantages: It hurts a lot. takes a lot of time till you start to see dreads (you will have a messy hair for at least a year). May damage a little bit of your hair if you are not careful enough.

NEGLECT / NATURAL / ORGANIC

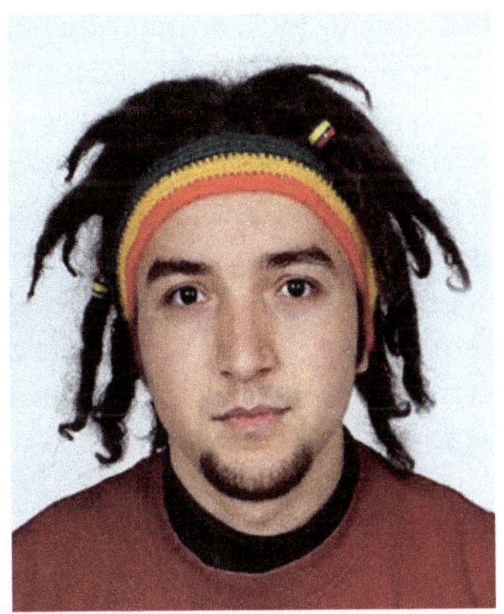

First thing you must know is that this is the best way to have healthy dreadlocks, but choosing the method is a personal choice.

Everyone is free to do whatever they want with their hair, choosing a "less natural" dreadlocks method will not make you any less than the all natural way dreadheads.

Second thing: many people when they hear "neglect method" they think that you neglect your hair in the way that you don't care about it or don't wash it..

WRONG.

Neglect method means: **no combing, not using any natural or chemical method to form the dreads and let the hair lock on itself with the minimum of help.**

How to do the Natural/ Neglect/ Organic method?

You basically don't do anything to your hair except **washing** it, your hair HAS to be clean. It takes from four months to one year (depending on your hair texture) your hair will then start to lock, at that time you will have to help sectioning your locked hair by separating the dreads at the roots.

It is important that you start sectioning your hair when it just start dreading or it will form huge *congos* (when two dreads or more lock together).

Do this separation regularly, anytime you feel like your hair needs it. It may sound like it's ripped, but it's normal you don't have to worry about it, the longer your dreads are growing, the less separation you will need to do.

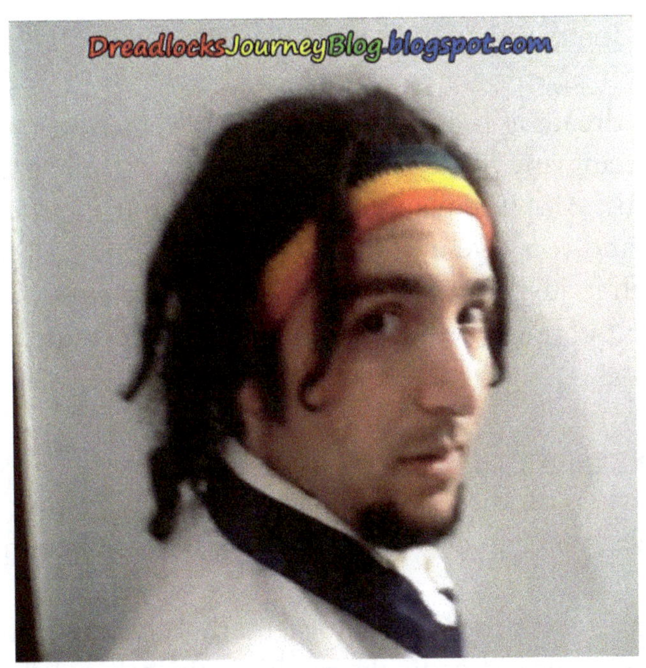

How often should I wash my "neglect" dreads??

You **wash your dreadlocks twice a week** and that's fine. Many Neglect people wash their hair less, like once a week, and that helps in forming the dreads faster, washing more than twice will slow down the dreading process, but it's up to you.

But you have to avoid any shampoo that leaves *residue* behind. Make sure you use **only natural residue free** dread Soap.

Maintaining neglect dreadlocks?

you don't have to do much really, Just separating the dreads and washing your hair.

But you may Moisturize your dreadlocks sometimes to avoid dryness, it helps keeping your hair healthy.

<u>**The golden word for Neglect dreadlocks is PATIENCE.**</u>

Yes, this dreading method needs a lot of patience, you will not be seeing any dreadlocks in the first year, only crazy messy hair. And if you set up your mind on using the neglect method and you give up before you reach your goal then it's not worth it, just some wasted time. So make sure you are patient enough to go all the way in. And believe me, it's really worth it.

<u>**Advantages of neglect dreadlocks.**</u>

It's an easy to do method, you don't need any help or experience, you can do it yourself. It is also the healthiest one.

I wouldn't say it's the only natural method because other than the chemical dreadlocks methods the other ones are natural too, but it's the most Natural one of them.

<u>**Disadvantages of neglect dreadlocks.**</u>

Takes a very long time so it needs a lot of patience, also the dreads are not all of the same size, and some people wouldn't like the "look" of their dreadlocks when they see different sizes on each dread. So if you care a lot about how your dreadlocks look, then this method is not for you.

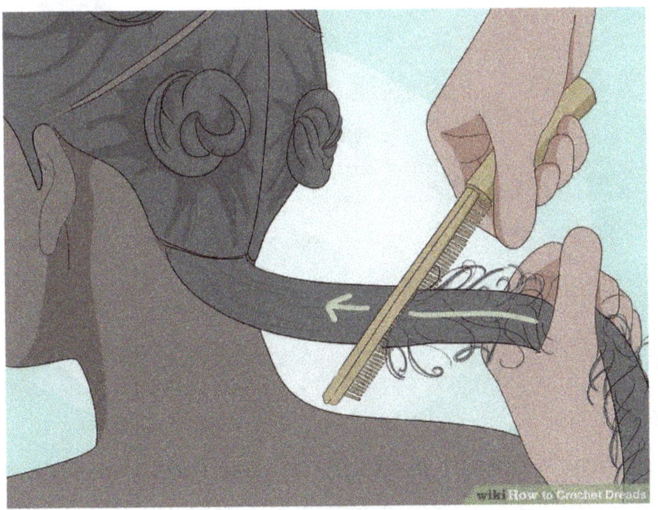

1 Courtesy of Wikihow.com

Backcombing method for dreadlocks is also a natural method of dreading IF you don't use any dread wax or product with it.
Backcombing works perfectly on all kind of hair, NO EXCEPTIONS even on very straight and smooth hair.. It's the method that proves that every human can have nice dreadlocks regardless of their background.

How to do the backcombing method?
First thing is that you section your hair in squares, you can choose from big or small depending on the dreads size you want, you may use rubber bands to secure your sections and take them off later.
then using a comb that has teeth close to each other like this one below:

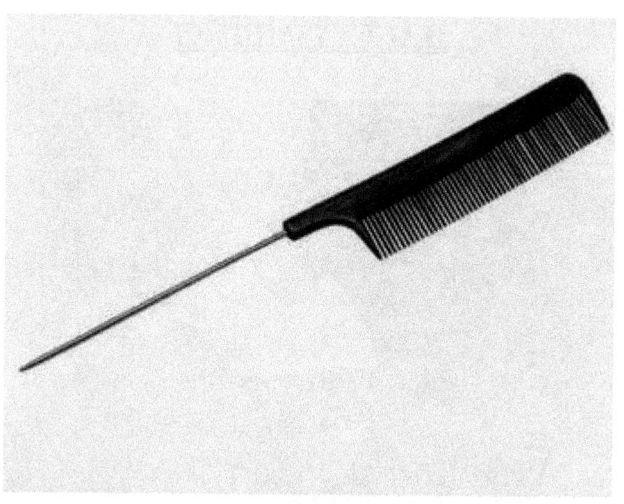

start combing the hair backwards, you begin from the root of the hair to the end of it inch by inch, meaning comb the first inch from the roots backwards then move to the inch above it and so on until you reach the tip of the sectioned hair. Do some palm rolling to help the locking process.

How often should I wash my backcombed dreads??
Just like we said in the neglect method in the previous section. Wash your dreadlocks twice a week and that's fine. It is a good idea if wash your hair less when you first backcomb it to give your newly dreads time to lock, like once a week. But remember.. Avoid any shampoo that
leave residue behind. Make sure you use only natural residue free dread Soap.

Maintaining backcombed dreadlocks?
Just like the neglected dreadlocks method, in backcombing.. you don't have to do much, Just separating the dreads and washing your hair. And some palm rolling sometimes
You may also Moisturize your dreadlocks sometimes.

<u>**Advantages of dreadlocks backcombing method:**</u>
while backcombing, you control the size of your dreads.
they mature faster than other methods.
backcombing works on all kind of hair especially straight
Caucasian and Asian hair.
It's almost an all natural method.

<u>**Disadvantages of dreadlocks backcombing method:**</u>
The backcombing process takes few hours.
Needs someone to help you with. it hurts sometimes.
You may lose some hair in the process.

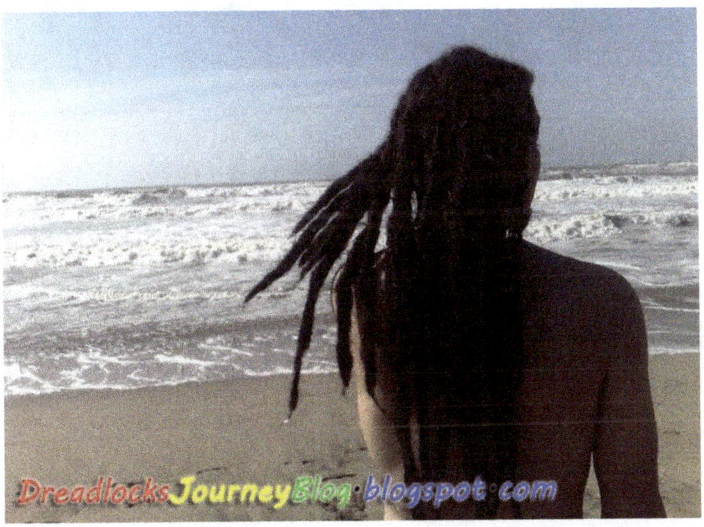

TWIST AND RIP

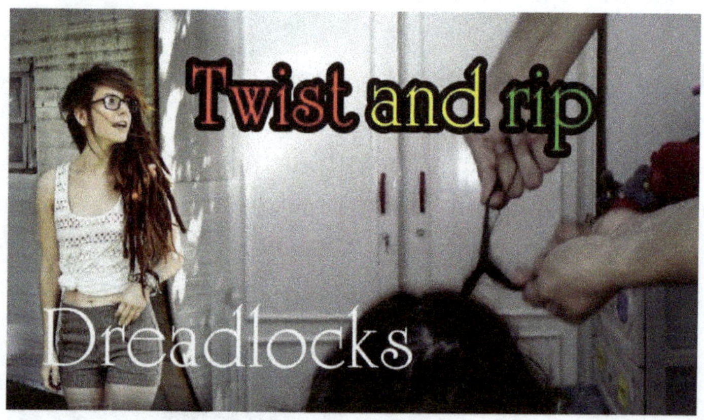

The twist and rip method to make dreadlocks is one of the most used methods, because it works on pretty much all types of hair and it's also an almost all natural dreading method **if** you don't use any dread wax with it.
But you have to know that once it's done and the dreads have locked, it's hard to unlock them.. So if you choose this method, you have to know that if you changed your mind about having dreadlocks you will go through a hard unlocking process.

How to do the twist and rip method?

First thing you do after washing your hair and drying it is
that you section your hair into square sections starting better
from the bottom of your hair, use rubber bands to secure
your sections then split the sectioned hair in two random
parts then rip until your reach the root, then twist again and
split the same section of hair in other two random parts and
rip again until the root, you will start to see knots
forming. keep twisting and ripping the whole section of hair
until you reach the tip of your hair.
But remember twist and rip or any other method you
use does not create dreadlocks, you are just helping to define
the size of your dreads by forming knots and keeping the
sectioned hair together, your hair will lock itself in a natural
process, but that will eventually take some time.
you might do some palm rolling as well, it doesn't do much
actually, it just keeps the section tidy.
keep twisting and ripping until you reach the tip of your hair,
as long as you can still hold hair between your fingers, then
use a rubber band on the tip of your hair as well.
When you finish twisting and ripping all your hair.. You do
not have to do anything else, just wait for your dreads to
mature.
Patience is the key to having beautiful healthy dreadlocks.

Twist and rip dreadlocks Maintenance

The twist and rip method just like any other dreadlocks
method, there is not much to be done, just washing your
hair, you may do some palm rolling if needed but you don't
have to. Sometimes the twist and rip locks get unlocked at
the end, you may need to re-twist them again.

You may also **Moisturize** your dreadlocks just like we said in the previous methods.

Washing your hair

You wash your dreadlocks twice a week just like we said before. Many people wash it less (when they first twist and rip) to speed up the locking process, but it's up to you. Also same warning about the use of a shampoo that leave residue behind. Make sure you use only natural residue free dread Soap.

Advantages

In the twist and rip method You control the size of your dreads. it's almost an all natural method (unless you use wax). your dreads look like real dreads the same day.

Disadvantages

doesn't work very well for some straight silky smooth hair. you may lose a little bit hair in the process. Hard to get it undone. may take time doing it and might hurt a little bit as well.

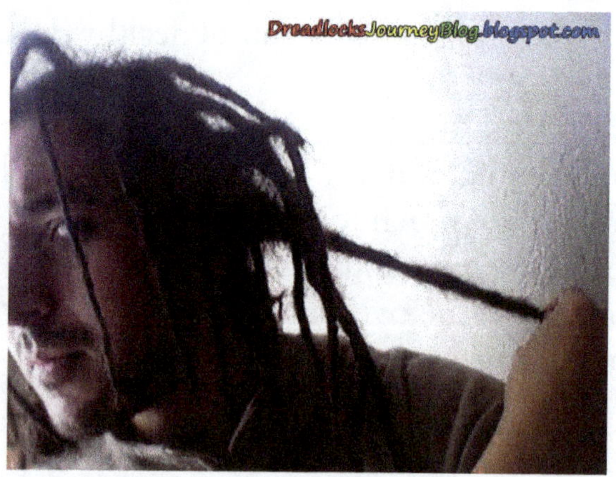

DREAD PERMING

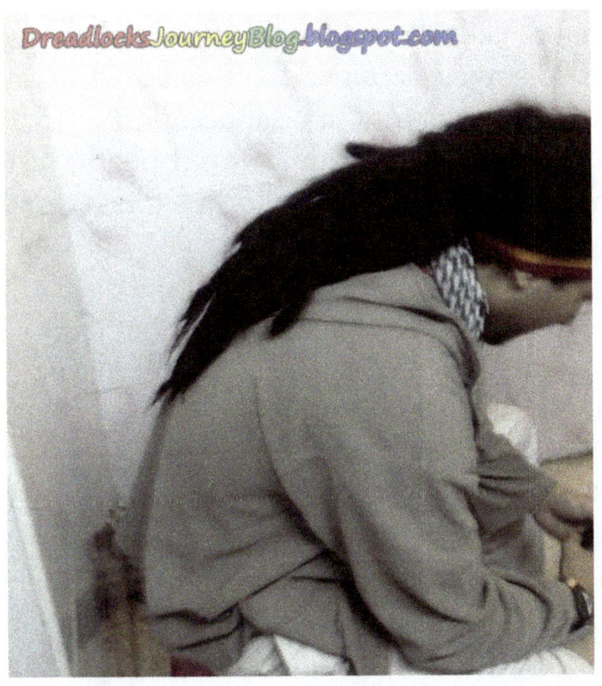

Dread perming would be the easiest way to have instant dreadlocks. Even if I am personally against this method, but I have to talk about it. After all, everyone is free to choose the dreading method that they want.

the dreadlocks perming method is mostly done in beauty salons, and it costs around $300 - $400. your hair will be exposed to chemical product that makes is frizzy, then bounded again and retreated with other chemical process to form the dreadlocks.

you will for sure have nice beautiful very well shaped dreadlocks instantly.

Although it is better when it's done by professionals, dread perming can also be done at home. Home perm kit cost around $10 - $20; and give similar results.

<u>Why people do dread perming to have dreadlocks?</u>
mostly people who are not patient and don't want to wait to have natural dreadlocks tend to do the dread perming method. Also some celebrities and models who want to have the "dreadlocks look" for a special occasion or for a photo session sometimes. Or sometimes some people just want to change their look without being bothered by everything else.

<u>How long does the dread perming take?</u>
the making of dread perming takes about 6 hours. And if done in a beauty salon, you will need maintenance appointments that take about two hours and costs about $200 every six months.

<u>Dread perming Advantages:</u>
after going out of the salon you will have dreadlocks.
after about six months it looks just like a natural grown dreadlocks
your dreads will have perfect shape and size
works on ALL hair even Asian straight silky

<u>Dread perming Disadvantages:</u>
The most un-natural dreading method
your hair will be exposed to chemical products
Risks if it's not done by professionals
Costs quiet a lot of money

WOOL METHOD

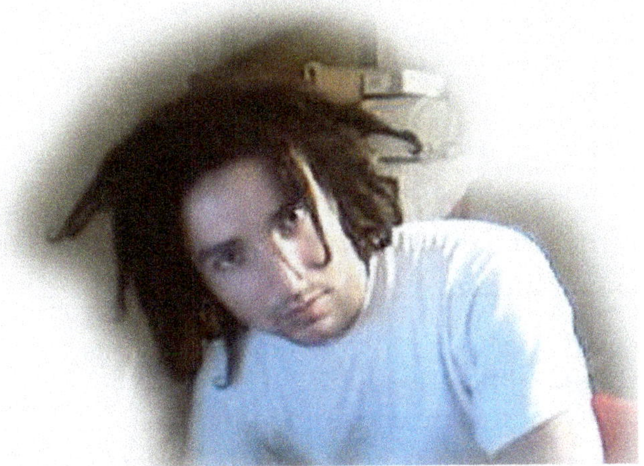

<u>What you need to know about Wool dreading:</u>
dreadlocks wool method is a lot similar to the neglect method, or you can say it's a neglect method with just a little help. If you are going to do this method you must be very patient, and I mean VERY patient. because it is one of the most "annoying" methods, and it takes a lot of time before you start to see real dreadlocks in your hair. You have to live with a crazy messy hair for at least a year, plus there is physical work you have to do almost every day.
For all those reasons, many people choose other dreading methods, but it's still one of the best and healthiest ones.

<u>**How to do it:**</u>

The basics of the wool method are very easy:

- Take a wool piece of clothing (sweater, hat or gloves or anything you have).
- Put it on your hair and rub it in circles for few minutes till you feel knots starting to form.
- You may rip it apart later to separately form your dreadlocks.
- Do this wool method process every time you have free time.
- Be patient and be ready to handle the pain.

<u>**Dreadlocks wool method Advantages:**</u>

Like the neglect dreadlocks, it's an all natural method, anyone can do it themselves no help needed, no tools (except a wool hat or something in wool).

<u>**Dreadlocks wool method disadvantages:**</u>

It hurts a lot while you are doing it. takes a lot of time till you start to see real dreads. You will have crazy messy hair for at least one year. You may lose a little hair in the process but it's ok it will grow back because the roots are not damaged or dead.

MAINTENANCE

<u>WASHING</u>

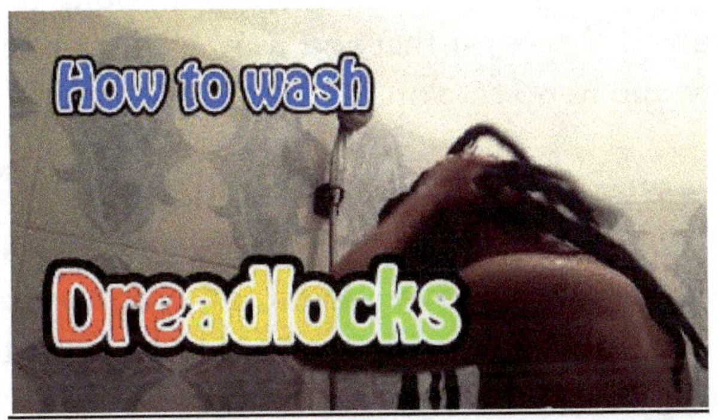

Washing dreadlocks is the number one dreads related issue that many people are confused about. Many think that in order to have dreadlocks you should stop washing your hair, while it is actually the other way around, if you want to have healthy clean dreadlocks you must wash them on a regular basis.

Clean dreadlocks mature fast while dirty hair is gross and makes your scalp itchy.

It is true that if you stop washing and brushing your hair it will also lock itself but in a very unhealthy way, locs will be filled with all kind of residue.

How long until I give my new dreads a first wash?

you do not have to wait at all, but it does help if you wait a little bit and allow your hair and scalp to get used to the new thing.

how much time you should wait depends on few factors:

* Your hair type
* How often do you usually wash your hair
* The method you used to make dreadlocks
* The climate where you live

So no one can tell you when to wash your young dreads except yourself, I suggest that you wait until your scalp starts to get itchy, the itchy-est you can handle.

How often should I wash my dreadlocks?

Same thing we said before, only YOU can decide, you can keep the same routine as you used to do before dreads or you can change it if you want, our bodies do adapt to anything new, so your scalp will get used to the new washing routine and will produce oils just as needed. So any washing routine would work just fine as long as it's not every day that is not good,

you can obviously shower your body without washing your dreadlocks.

Shampoo and soap

there are many shampoos and soaps available. But what works well for one may not work well for the other, that's why it's better if you read reviews, ask your dreadhead friends try many types of shampoos and soaps and see which one works best for you. As long as it's residue free. you can even make your own soap if you want.

<u>**My personal dreadlocks washing routine:**</u>
you may do just as I do or you can do your own, the keys
are: residue free shampoo, good rinsing and good drying.

- I first get my hair wet and give my scalp a gentle massage
- Then I put some of my shampoo on my palms and rub it all over my scalp (I don't use it on my dreads because that will happen later, also if your dreads are new be gentle with the rubbing)
- I get under the shower, the shampoo becomes bubbly and I rub it all over my scalp and dreads very well (massage carefully if your dreads are new)
- once I feel that I shampooed all my hair I proceed to rinsing
- I set the shower to the strongest mode and let water run through my dreads (the more you stay under water the better)
- I squeeze my dreads to get new clean water runing through them again
- I repeat the rinsing and squeezing until I feel it's enough
- I turn off the shower and start squeezing my dreads to get all the water out

Once I feel that I can't get any more water out and my
dreads stopped dripping I proceed to drying.

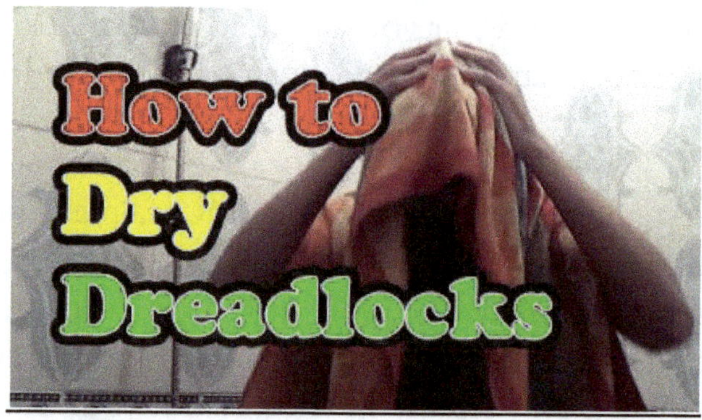

Drying dreadlocks is one of the most annoying routines for any dreadhead, because it's time and energy consuming. Unlike washing dreadlocks that takes only 10 to 30 minutes, and no matter what you do, drying your dreadlocks will take hours.

Here are few points to know about drying dreadlocks:

1- Wash your dreadlocks early:
First thing you should know is that it's better that you wash your dreadlocks early in the day if you can, the earlier the better, that way you will allow them to air dry before you go to bed, it's not recommended that you sleep with wet dreadlocks.

2- Drying starts from the shower:
right after washing your dreads, proceed to squeezing them very well to get as much water out as you could.

I do **not** recommend doing "head bangs" because shaking your head **could be dangerous**, but if you want to do that, just be careful and don't shake too hard, it does help a little bit in getting the water to the tips of your dreads.

3- Using Towels:

you will mostly need two towels or more, because dreadlocks suck a lot of water in. rub the towel on your head and dreads, just like you used to do with your long hair before dreadlocks.
wrap your dreads in the towel and squeeze them.

4- Blow drying:

be careful while using the blow dryer, do not set it to maximum heat (you don't want to fry your dreads from outside) and don't apply it on one spot for a very long time either. Same things you would actually do with unlocked hair. You may put a towel on your dreads and make some kind of a tunnel and blow dry them while they're inside the towel , it helps trapping the hot air in, that way the hot hair will circulate inside and won't get wasted all over the room.. and therefore more chance to get dry dreadlocks faster.

5- Sleeping with wet dreads:

If you have to sleep with dreads that are not 100% dry, put a towel on your pillow and spread your dreads all over it.

Different people will have different results, depending on the hair type, the size and length of dreads, and the weather where one lives, people living a hot places are luckier than the ones living in cold humid areas.

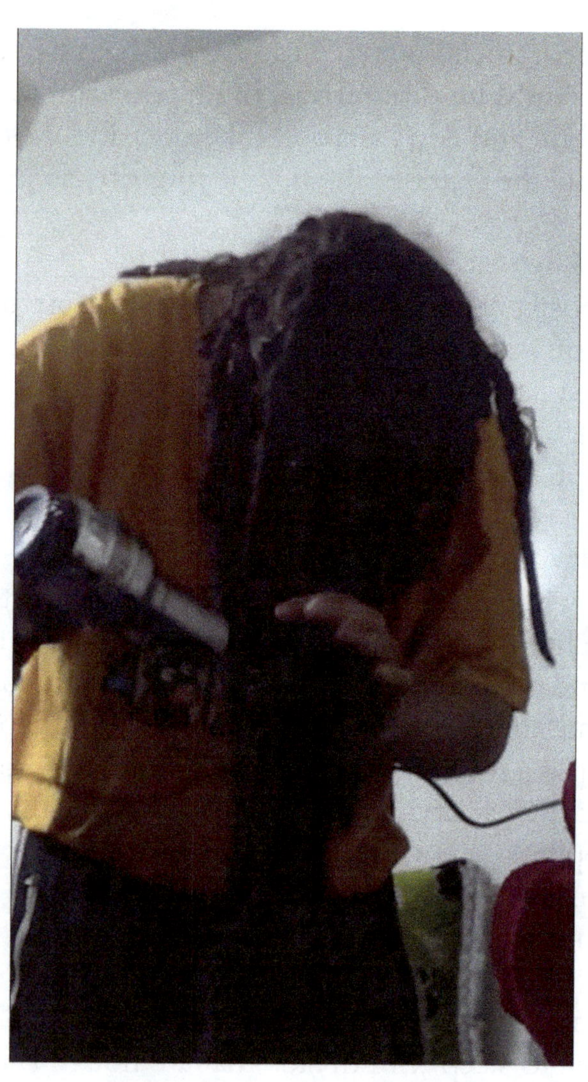

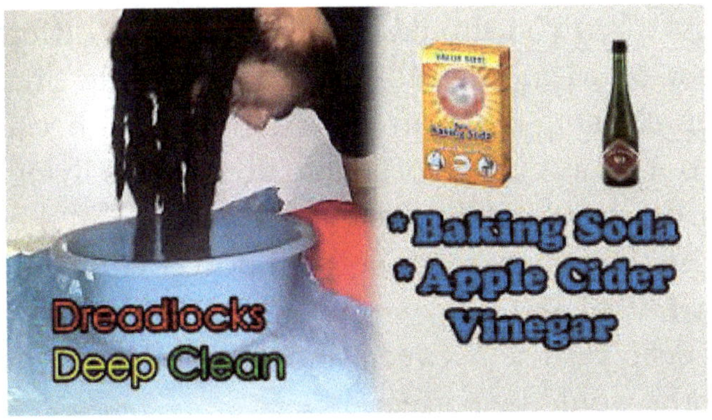

Every now and then, you will need to deep clean your dreadlocks. not only because regular washing is not enough to clean your dreads from the inside out, but also for the other benefits that a deep cleanse have. You will literally feel the change once you have soaked your dreads in a deep clean recipe, you will notice that your locks are a lot lighter. Remember, no matter what residue free shampoo you are using for your dreadlocks, it is never 100% residue free

The first deep cleanse of your baby dreads:
basically your baby dreads will not need deep cleaning for a while, washing would be enough, because you still don't have any build up yet.
But at some point you will notice that washing is not enough, you will also notice that your dreads are getting easily kind of stiff some time after washing them. Just keep an eye on your dreads and with time you will know when they need a deep cleaning.

How often to deep clean dreadlocks?

Same as above, keep an eye on your dreads and you will know how often you should do it, because it is different from a person to another, for example very tight dreads will need deep cleaning more often than loose ones because build up does not go away with washing, dreadheads living in windy or hot areas tend to have more build up in their dreads.. Also it depends on the shampoo you use, and many other stuff.

Ideally a deep cleanse between once a month and once every two months would be perfect

How to deep clean dreadlocks?

What most (if not all) dreadheads use to deep clean dreads is the Baking Soda soak. (Baking Soda is also called bicarbonate of soda), it is famous for its cleaning benefits and also available and cheap.

The most basic dreadlocks deep clean recipe:

- Bowl / Sink / Bucket...: Anything that could help you soak your dreads for about 30 minutes. Make sure all your hair will sink in water, and try to find a comfortable position.
- Warm water: fill the bowl or sink or whatever you are using with hot water, as hot as you can stand but not too hot.
- Baking soda / Bicarbonate of Soda: add few table spoons to the warm water, how much to add depends on how much water you are using.. just don't use too much until it builds up at the bottom.
- Stir very well
- Take out any beads or accessories left in your dreads

- Soak your dreads in the bowl or bucket
- Massage your scalp
- Squeeze your dreads to get water out and soak them again
- Keep your dreads soaked for about 30 minutes along with squeezing and massaging
- Rinse your dreadlocks very well afterwards

Now it is time for the apple cider vinegar:

Please note that you need Apple cider vinegar after baking soda because it will balance the PH of your hair:

- You can either re-sink your dreads in a bowl filled with apple cider vinegar and water
- Or you can use a spray bottle and spray apple cider vinegar all over your dreads.
- Rinse your dreads very well again.
- Proceed to washing your hair with shampoo like you usually do.

You will notice that your dreads are lighter and cleaner than usual.

PALM ROLLING

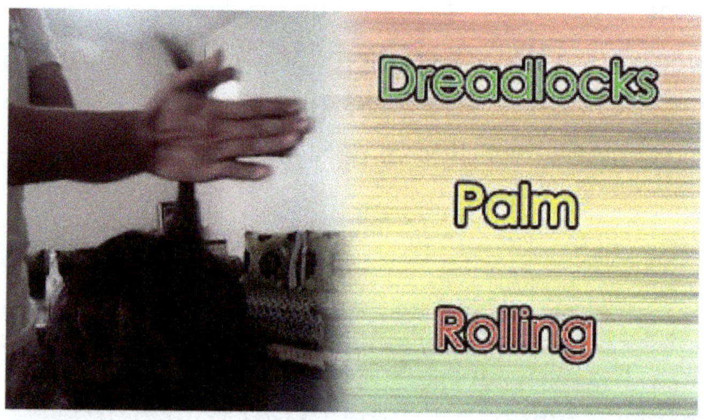

Palm Rolling dreadlocks means simply grabbing the dread between the base of your palms and rubbing it back and forth, along with compressing it with your palms.

Many people believe that palm rolling helps the knots to compress and tighten and therefore to become dreadlocks. I personally from my own experience don't think so, I have done it when I started my first set and it really didn't do anything to my dreadlocks, It gives you an instant neat look for your dreads but that doesn't last very long since the hair does not actually lock inside the dread, it just lay on the dread from the outside for a while or until you wash your dreads.

But palm rolling dreadlocks could be useful in some cases:

*** If you are using wax or cream:** I do not recommend using wax on dreadlocks, any kind of wax, but I don't judge people who do use it, especially organic wax. In this case palm rolling really helps a lot. It gets all the frizzy hair to stick with the dread and gives dreadlocks a more mature look.

*** When you are backcombing or twisting your hair:** because the dread is still in the process of forming, palm rolling while backcombing or twisting really helps, it does get all the messy hair inside the dread before being back combed by the brush or getting twisted in, that way it stays inside and helps tightening the dread.

*** The ends of dreads:** palm rolling can also help locking the tip of your dreads when they loosen up, because in that area it is easy to get the hair to lock

*** In the lumps and bumps phase:** when your dreadlocks go through the shrinkage phase (if they ever do), palm rolling them after washing could help speeding up the process of uniforming.

Again that is just my own experience. The outcome will be different from hair texture to another, but you may try palm rolling and see how it works for your dreadlocks. Sometimes I do it just because I like to play with my dreads
But Remember, no matter why you are palm rolling your dreads, never do it too hard and never do it close to the roots, you may break your hair and hurt your scalp.

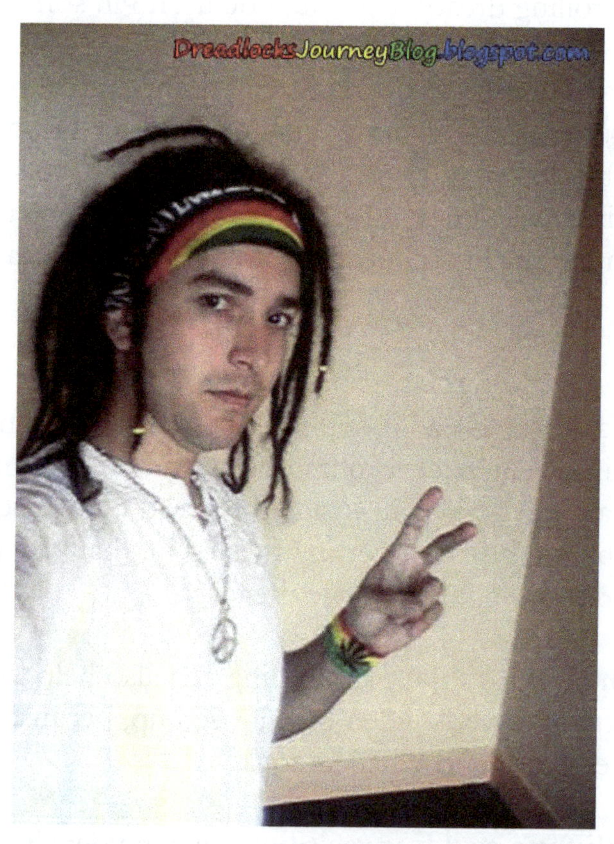
DreadlocksJourneyBlog.blogspot.com

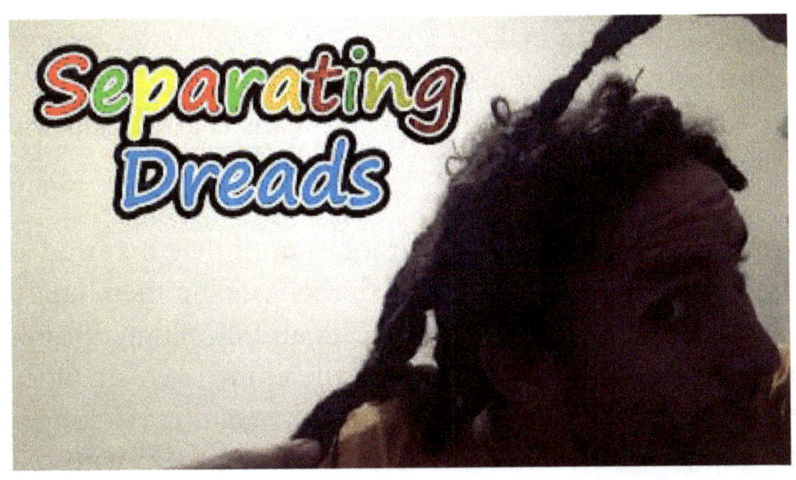

Dreads will always try to grow together at the roots, especially if you are using the neglect method. So if you want to avoid that, if you don't want to have any "congos" or very thick locks, which some other people would love to have, you should just separate them regularly.
Simply grab the two dreads (or more) that are conjoined together, and pull them apart from each other all the way to the roots.. you do not have to separate your dreads all the way to the scalp, as this may in some cases cause some dread thinning at the roots with time.
you will hear some cracking hair sound, but that's ok don't worry about it.

Separating dreadlocks is a process that all dreadheads do, no matter what method they used to have dreadlocks, even dreadheads who want congos they still want to control how many dreads are going to be in every new formed one.

So if you are planning to have dreadlocks, be prepared, along with washing and drying, separating your dreads is a routine you will have to get used to.
It is better that you make it a habit, every other day, play with your locks by separating them.
Note that the best time to separate dreads is after the shower before they are 100% dry.

If you were not separating your locks until they matured and congos have already been formed, then pulling them apart will become very hard.. At that point and if pulling doesn't work.. the best way to split a thick dread into two smaller dreads is to brush it out and re-dread it again.(It is a long and annoying process but it's better than cutting them with scissors)
But if you don't want to put that much time and effort in brushing out and starting over again then the only way to separate a congo is using scissors.
But scissors must be the last choice, and it's better that you get someone else to do the cutting for you.

LOOSE HAIR TOOL / LATCH HOOK

The loose hair tool for dreadlocks looks like the following:

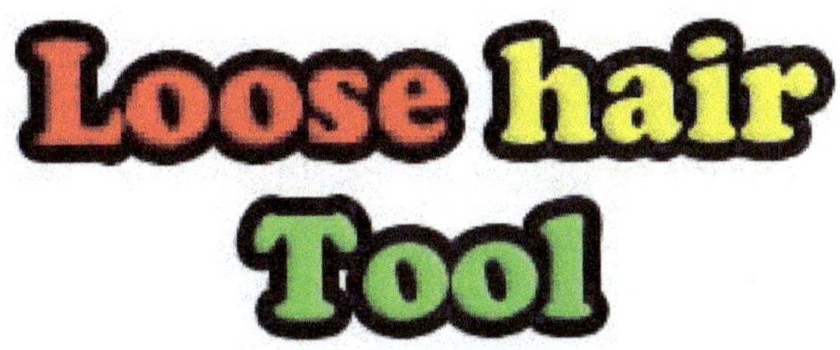

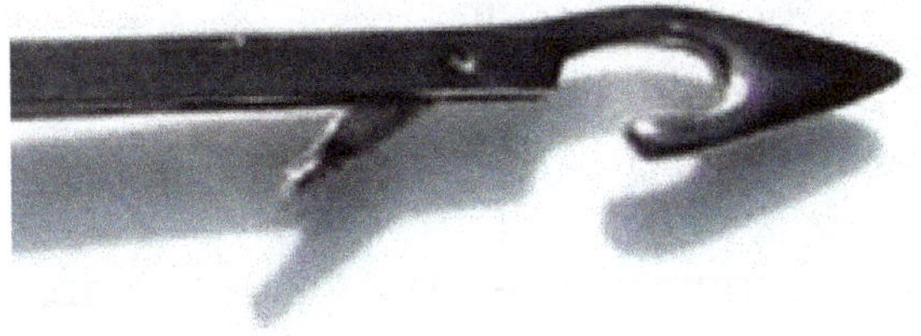

The loose hair can be a very annoying problem to people with dreadlocks, dealing with it is one of the reasons why dreadlocked people invented maintenance. The Crochet hook is one way that could help you get all the loose hair inside the dread, but crocheting dreadlocks required a little bit of skills, I'm not saying it's hard but using the lose hair tool is much easier, anyone can use it on their dreadlocks with no problem.

You can find this dreadlocks loose hair tool in dreads stores, or you can get a latch hook at any craft store.

How to use it:

A)-On the root:

1. roll the loose hair between your fingers
2. find the dread that the loose hair belong to (or the closest dread it could fit in)
3. roll the loose hair between your fingers and thumb to make a small hair ball
4. measure how long in the dread would the loose hair take to fit entirely inside
5. insert the loose hair tool inside the dread slightly above the point you measured (to make sure that the loose hair wouldn't come out when you pull out the latch hook)
6. slide the tool all the way in the center of the dread until you touch your scalp
7. pull it out, hook the hair ball and close the latch
8. pull it back inside the dread until it comes out

and that's it, all the loose hair is now inside the dread and going to lock with no problem.

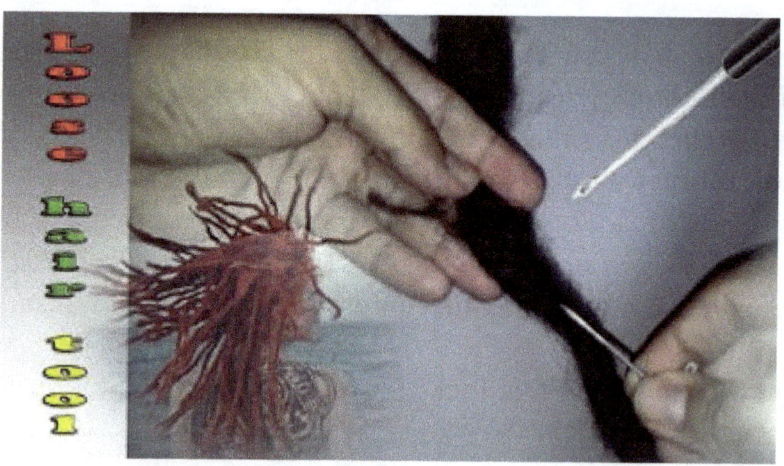

B)-Anywhere along the dread:

You pick all the loose hair around the dread but only in 2 inches area, otherwise it's not going to be easy to get it inside. The rest is similar to how you use it on the root, pull inside and pull out at the base of the loose hair, hook the hair and pull it back.

You can also use it at the tip of the dread to get the hair back inside and give the tip of your dread a nice round shape.
This is one way among others that can ensure you a good dreadlocks maintenance.

<u>For thin dreads:</u>
It is the same procedure, except that instead of getting all the loose hair inside the dread, you keep getting it in and out until it fits in
For thin dreads you should be careful about the size of any tool you uses on them.
There are other issues you need to be aware of while using a dreadlocks loose hair tool, a crochet hook or any other maintenance tool:
1)- **It is very normal to have loose hair before your dread mature**, there is nothing to panic about
2)- **Do NOT use any maintenance tool unless you really have to**, using tools on your dreads all the time may create holes and might do some damages.
3)- **While using any tool on your dreadlocks, use it gently**, do not pull hard, to not be violent to your dreads.
4)- **Be patient**, make peace with the fluffy frizzy loose hair around your dreadlocks, it is normal to have loose hair all the time that will eventually end up locking itself.

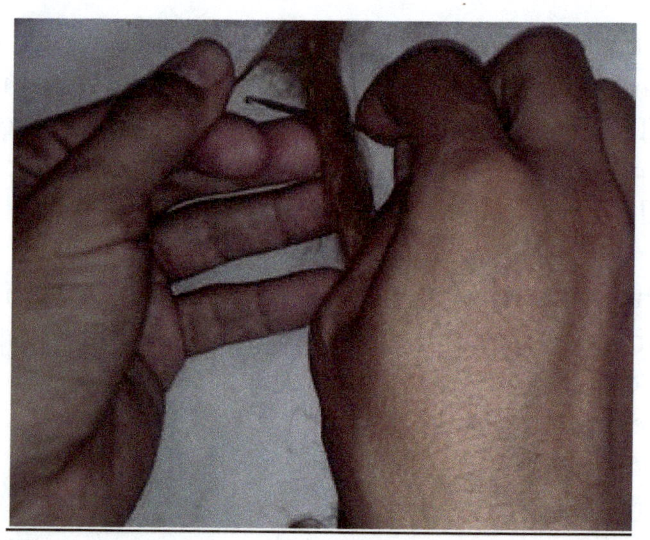

CROCHETING

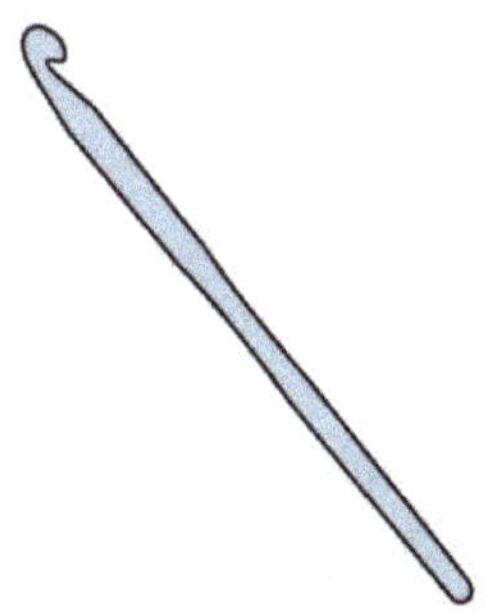

There is a huge debate about using crochet hook to start or to maintain dreadlocks. Just like everything else. While some see it a great tool that gives great instant results, others believe that it can damage your dreads.
I personally think that each case is different, different people will have different outcomes, because it depends on how do you crochet your dreads, how tight are they, do you crochet at the roots where being rough is not recommended, or at the tips where it is ok to do pretty much anything (because no matter the damages you did you could easily cut them off).
So the choice is yours, if you decide to crochet your locs here is how you do it:

1-Choose the smallest size you could find:
that way any bad move you do will have the least impact on your dreads, bigger hooks might even create holes in your dreads.

2-For starting dreadlocks:

Proceed just as you would do with the backcombing or twist and rip method (sectioning, securing your sections, backcombing or twisting) then move on to crocheting just as you would do for maintenance.

3-For maintenance:
- Insert the crochet hook through the section of hair about 1/4 in (0.64 cm) from where the section meets the scalp. Get a few strands of hair on the hook from the other side of the section.
- Next, carefully pull the hook with the hairs on it back through the section of hair. Make sure that the hairs don't slip off as you do this. If they do, you will need to repeat the step to get a few hairs on the hook again.
- Repeat the process, After you have pulled the first few hairs through your section, do the same thing over again. Insert the hook into the dread about 1/4 in (0.64 cm) down from where you started, hook a few strands of hair, and pull them through the section again. Keep going until you reach the bottom of the section. (If you notice hairs poking out of a section of the dread once you reach the bottom, simply go back to that section and use the crochet hook to grasp them and pull them through)
- After you finish locking the dread, go back over it at least 1 time with the crochet hook to tighten it up. Push the crochet hook into the dread about halfway and pull it back quickly a few times while keeping the hook inside of the dread. Then, move down the section about 1/4 in (0.64 cm) and repeat.

4-for blunting the tips:

- Hold the crochet hook parallel to the end of your dreadlock. Grasp a dreadlock about 2 in (5.1 cm) from the end and hold your crochet hook next to it. Position the crochet hook so that it is parallel to your dreadlock and the hook is beside the end of the dreadlock.
- Push the hook into the dreadlock and out the end. Insert the hook into the dreadlock about 1 in (2.5 cm) from the end. Push the hook into your dreadlock going down towards the end of the dreadlock. Bring it out at the end of your dreadlock so that you can grasp a few hairs with the hook when you pull it back through.
- After you push the hook out the bottom of the dreadlock, pull it back up into the dreadlock to bring a few stray hairs into the dreadlock. Do this quickly and don't pull the hairs all the way out of the dreadlock where you inserted the hook. Bring them into the dreadlock so that they will be hidden.
- Continue to quickly push the hook in and out of the dreadlock, going past the end, and pulling hairs back up and into the dreadlock. After a few minutes of this, the end will look round-ish.

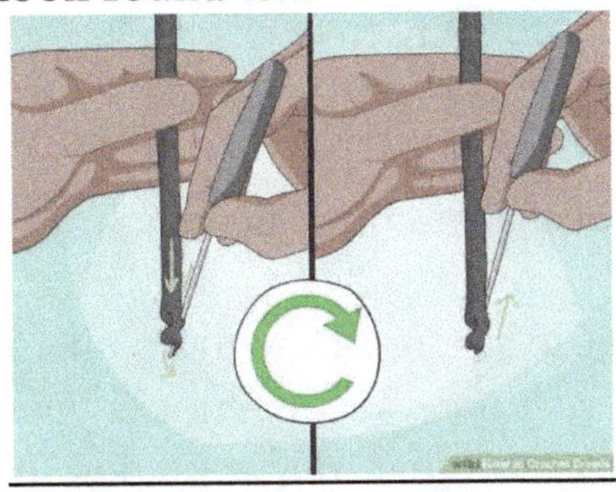

2courtesy of wikihow.com

SEA SALT SPRAY

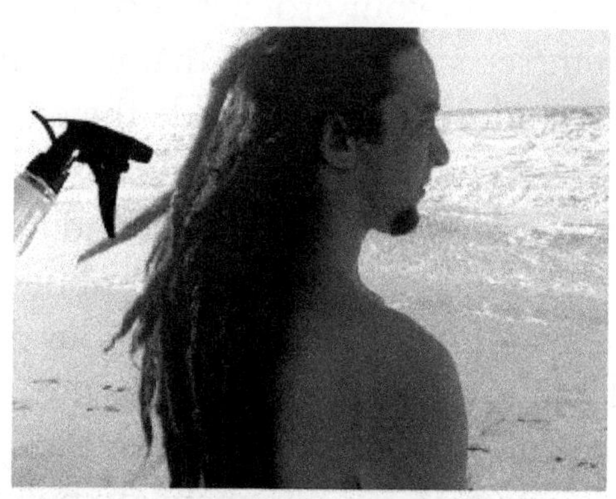

Sea salt is amazing for dreadlocks, it is a process accelerator because it makes the hair frizzy and knotty and dry too. Therefore it increases the formation of locks. it is not only perfect for young dreads, but also for lose hair on fully matured dreadlocks.

You can get the benefits of sea salt by swimming regularly in the ocean, if you do not live by the ocean or you just cannot swim for any other reason, you can still have the same effects by making a sea salt spray.

to make a sea salt spray for dreadlocks:

You will need:

Warm water

Warm only because it takes less time for the salt to dissolve

Sea salt

It is better to use a pure salt with no chemical additives, you only want the salt on your dreadlocks you do not need to have other products that might build in inside your dreads

<u>**Spray bottle**</u>

the best and easy-to-use way to apply the salt all over your dreads

How to make a sea salt spray:

- Add just enough salt to water, it does not matter how much since eventually you only want the salt, the water will evaporate, but adding too much may just clog your spray tube and that would be annoying.
- stir very well till the salt dissolves completely in the water.

That's it! your sea salt spray bottle is ready to use on your dreads.

<u>**Where to apply it**</u>

- Spray everywhere on your young dreads because the knots are still forming.
- For mature dreadlocks you may just spray on loose hair spots like on the tips or the new growth.

<u>**Important:**</u>

1- While spraying avoid your eyes and your hair scalp, having much salt on your scalp might be irritating.

2- If you are just starting to use sea salt it is better that you start spraying for short period of time before showering, because you don't know your hair reaction to salt.

3- If your hair is of the dry type avoid sea salt, as it may dry it more and that would damage it.

Notes:

Some people add lemon juice to the sea salt bottle, and that increases the dryness, but be careful if your hair gets easily dry. You may try and see the result yourself before deciding either to use it or not.

Other people add essential oils, but actually essential oils do the opposite effect of salt, it will only reduce the effectiveness of salt.

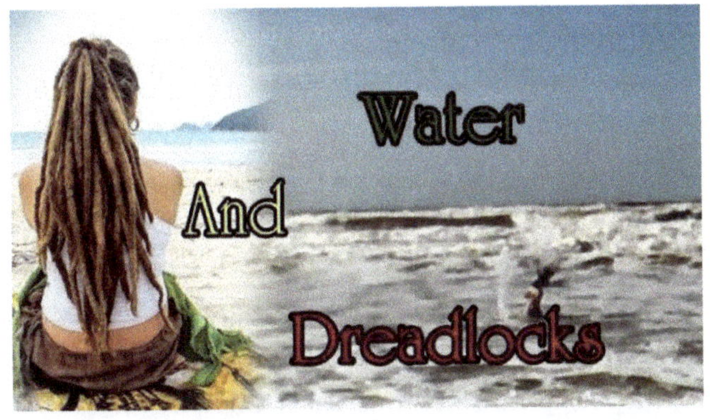

whenever summer approaches, there are some common questions about dreadlocks that come up, especially for new dreaded people. the most common one is about swimming with dreadlocks. here is what you should know about this issue.

1-To swim with dreadlocks is completely fine, especially in the ocean because salty water helps your dreads to mature and to tighten up. most dreadlock experts suggest swimming in the ocean for a better and faster dreading process. Thus, it is a good idea to let the salty water dry in your dreadlocks before washing them. Or you can make your own homemade salt water spray as an alternative to swimming.

2-if your dreads are less than 1 month old, it's better that you avoid swimming too often, if you can't resist the swimming temptation, you may use a swimming cap, or if you don't have one, at least use rubber bands at the root and the tip of each dread.

3-It is ok to also swim in pools. the Chlorine doesn't hurt your dreads as long as you rinse them well right after you get out of water then wash them as soon as possible.
Notice that in some hotel pools some people may jump in with sun tan oils on, that makes the water oily, it's better if you avoid swimming or use a swim cap.

4-if you're swimming with dreadlocks in their first few months, you may notice some loose hair afterwards, it's ok, it does not mean that your dreads are falling apart, just deal with it with a loose hair tool or a crochet hook

5-Make sure to dry your dreads after showering, do not sleep with them wet or put them in a hat, if you had no choice but sleeping with wet dreads, spread them along to allow them air drying.

6-it is better to not swim in lakes and rivers without a swimming cap, no matter how clean they look, or if you have to then make sure to rinse your dreads very well afterwards.

<u>Bottom line:</u> swim, have fun, but wash your dreads, rinse and dry them.

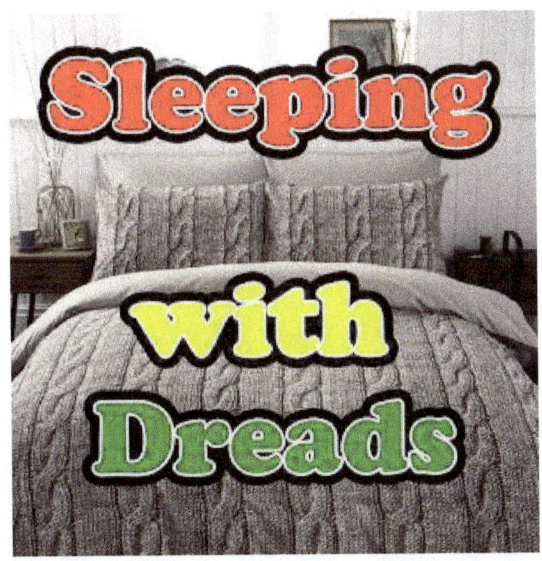

There are no rules to how to properly sleep with dreadlocks, most dreadheads just sleep without thinking of what to do and what not to do, but when you first start your dreadlock journey you always tend to over think about everything, you want to do everything right and not to miss any kind of maintenance.

Anyway, you may use some of these tips:

1- Clean your pillow and sheets from any visible lint or dust, dreadlocks are like magnet to dust, you don't want them to catch anything while you're sleeping.

2- You may put a wool cover on your pillow to encourage the knotting, especially if your dreads are young, a lot of knotting will happen when you sleep.

3- You may also make a dread bun on the top of your head, it is more comfortable than having them tied up in the back when it feels like sleeping on a big lump.

<u>4-</u> Putting your dreads in a T shirt prevents them from getting in your face while you are sleeping and also keeps them free to move around, unlike when they are tied up or in a bun.

<u>5-</u> Always try to avoid sleeping with damp dreads but if you have to then put a towel on your pillow, and spread your dreads all over it.

<u>6-</u> If your dreads are young you may sleep with a loose wool hat, it would help the dreads knotting and it's also comfortable to sleep with.

Eventually you will end up sleeping with your dreads the same way you use to sleep with your normal hair and there's nothing wrong with that, but sleeping on your dreads in the same way every night may cause some of them to become flat.

REMOVING DREADLOCKS

First of all, think again before deciding to remove your dreads. especially if you didn't reach that stage where you can see long rope-like beautiful dreadlocks, it's really an experience that you do not want to miss.

But I understand if you still want to proceed, people have their reasons for doing so, I had to remove my first set of dreads because it was not appropriate for the job I was applying for.

Cutting off:

the easiest fastest way to remove your locs is to simply cut them few inches to the roots (the area that generally haven't locked yet).

Brushing out:

Now that's a real long time-consuming process. It is even more painful when the dreadlocks are long and tight, so it is better to have at least one person to help you out.

You will need:
- Warm water
- Knitting or sewing needles
- Hair brushes
- Hair conditioner
- De-tangler if possible

How to proceed:
- Soak your dreads in warm water.
- Rub the hair conditioner into your dreadlocks

- Once the dreadlocks are wet and conditioned start pulling them apart with a knitting or sewing needle starting from the tips of course
  (slip the needle into the edge of a dread near the tip, push it into a loop and then slowly pull the loop out. You're going to only pull a small amount at a time. It's like as if you are brushing your hair, but with just one tooth at a time).

- Re-apply warm water and hair conditioner when needed, because since it is a very long process your dreads might dry out and trust me you don't want that extra pain.

- The more you get close to the root of your dreads the more careful you must be, your scalp needs to be treated with extra care.

- Do not freak out when you see a lot of loose hair falling out, it is just the regular amount of hair that would fall out when your hair was un-dreaded, except that your dreads kept it inside.

- Be extra careful with needles or any sharp tool you are using.

STYLING DREADLOCKS

WRAPPING DREADLOCKS

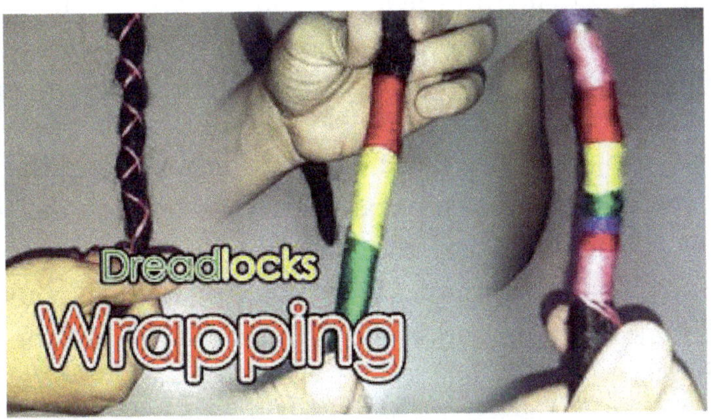

Dreadlocks wrapping is the first thing that many dreadheads cannot wait to do as soon as they are done with starting their dreads. However, just like anything related to the health and safety of your dreadlocks, there are few points you need to know.

When should I start wrapping my dreadlocks?

The best would be that you wait until your dreads are fully matured before starting any sort of decoration or accessorizing, let them do their thing, the process is long and needs a lot of patience. And wrapping them will slow down the locking process.

But, you can still wrap your less-than-mature dreads as long as you do not keep them wrapped for a long time. I would suggest a day maximum, like if you are having a party, going to an event or something like that, or if you just want to take some beautiful pictures of your decorated locks.

Types of wrapping:

there are actually no rules and you can wrap your dreads however you want, but there are two major types of dread wraps that you can play with and invent your own style:

Criss-cross wraps: these open string wraps are the best for young dreadlocks, because they do not "choke" or squeeze the dread and allow it to breath, but if you leave the strings long enough on your young dreads, your hair will lock on them and it will be hard to take out the strings afterwards.

How to do Criss-cross wraps: you simply do it by making a knot on the point where you want to start wrapping, then criss-crossing, or kind of braiding the two parts of the strings with the dread, until you reach the desired final point then secure with a knot.

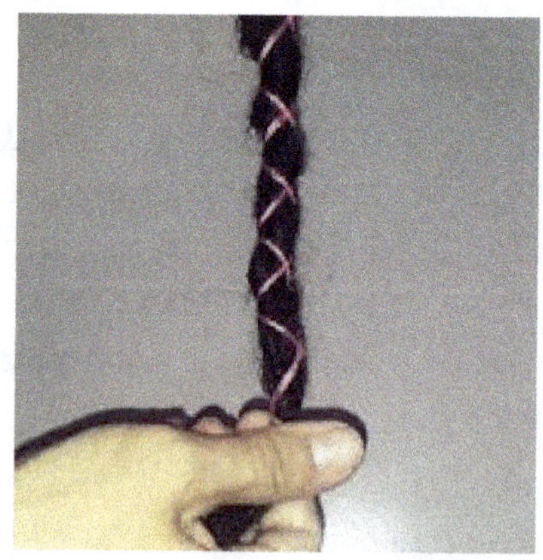

<u>Solid thread wraps:</u> these are not recommended for young locks as they choke the dread and stop it from locking and may cause weak spots. But if you decide to wrap your young dreads do not leave them for too long as we said and also try to make your wraps loose, do not squeeze the dread.

<u>How to do solid thread wraps:</u> It can simply be done by making a knot at the top of the desired area, then wrapping the thread around the dread without leaving any "free spaces". You may use more than one color by attaching new thread every time you are done with one color, or by attaching threads of all the colors you want from the beginning and start wrapping using one color at a time.. then secure with a knot at the end.

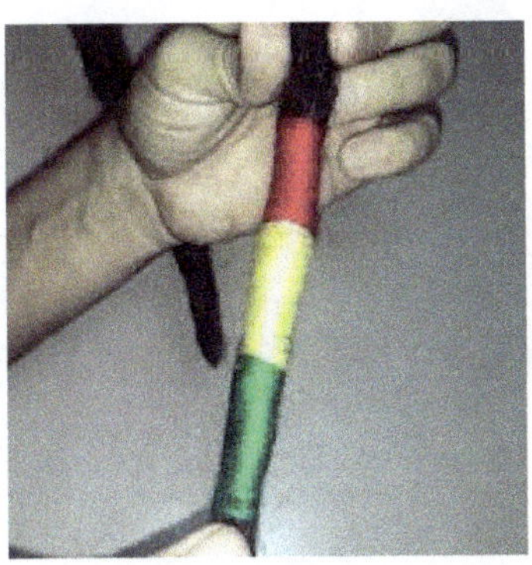 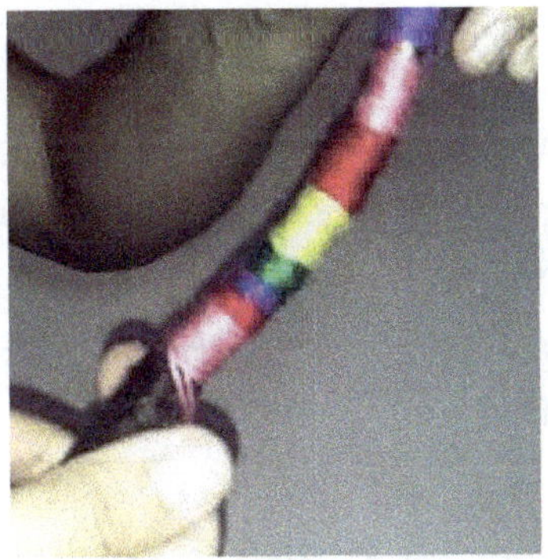

BEADS

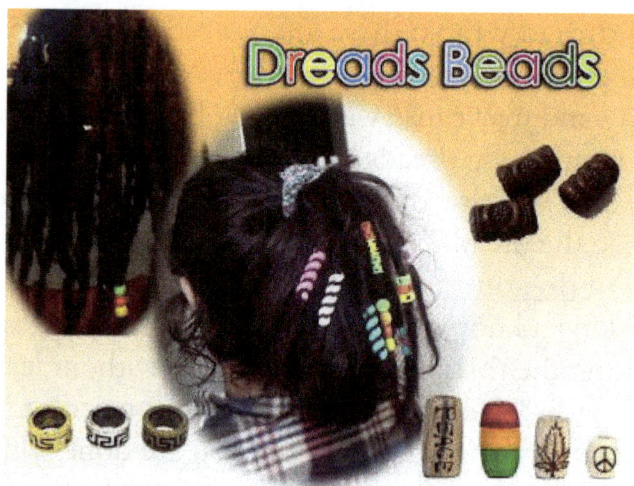

As mentioned in the "wrapping" section, decoration and accessories are one of the most important stages that many dreadheads are looking forward to.

For some people it's even one of the reasons that attracted them to start a dreadlocks journey in the first place. Just like the dreadlocks wrapping that we talked about previously, there is nothing wrong with decorating your dreads with beads as long as you know everything about how to and when to use beads.

Beads on young dreadlocks:

I must say it again, it is not recommended to put beads on young dreads, because dreads should be left alone to do their things. But you can still decorate your young dreads with beautiful beads as long as you don't leave them on for a long time..

(If you leave beads on your young dreads for very long time your hair might start locking on them and then it would be hard to take them off, same as in wrapping)

Washing and deep cleaning dreadlocks:
Whenever you proceed to washing or deep cleaning your dreads, you should take all the beads off, leaving the beads on will eventually cause some build up in the hidden areas, also those hidden areas won't be cleaned properly which is not cool

What beads to use:
There are many kinds of beads to choose from: glass, plastic, wood, metal... you may use any one you want, I have never heard of anyone having problems using a special kind of beads.. maybe if you're allergic to one of the ingredients you might better avoid that kind of beads. I personally like wooden beads. I also have had metal ones, but I was never crazy about beads, maybe couple here and there and that's it.

DREAD BUN

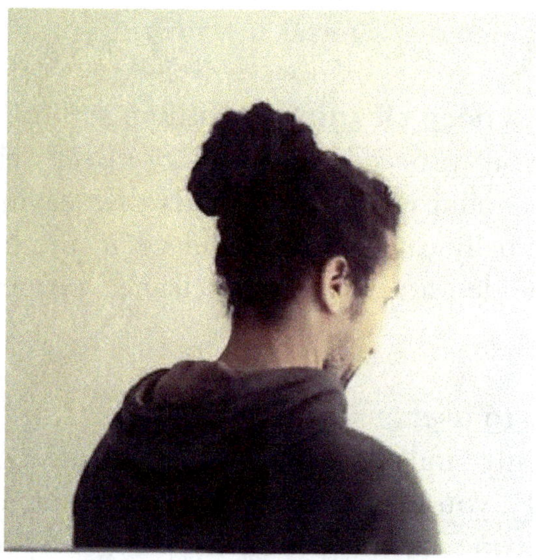

You have your long beautiful dreadlocks now, you are doing all kind of dreads maintenance: washing them properly, drying them.. now it's time to think about styles and how to wear them.

There are several choices as to how to style your dreadlocks, this section is only about one of them, making a dread bun. But there are other ways to wear your dreads such as tying them in the back or make a ponytail or even wearing a hat. There are also no rules to "how to make a dread bun" you can play around with your dreads and invent your own style as long as your dreads are long enough to form a bun. Or you can just watch YouTube videos and see how other dreadheads make dread buns and get inspired.

Style 1:

I have seen many dreadheads doing it this way

- First put your dreads in a high ponytail using an elastic headband, this will allow you to gather them all into a single bunch.
- Then twist your dreads from roots to ends while forming a circle around the headband.
- Secure your bun by tucking the tips of your dreads under the headband

Style 2:

This is the easiest one to do, just get your dreads only half way through the headband, it will automatically form a bun, you will still have your dreads down a little bit but that way they will be less annoying and they cannot reach your face.

Style 3:

This one works only for very long dreads, and will need some practice, it is similar to dread bun in style one I mentioned above but without using a headband.
Twist your dreads, form a circle, and secure just by tucking each dread under the bun you are forming. It may not look very secured but I have seen people doing it without any headbands and it doesn't fall off.

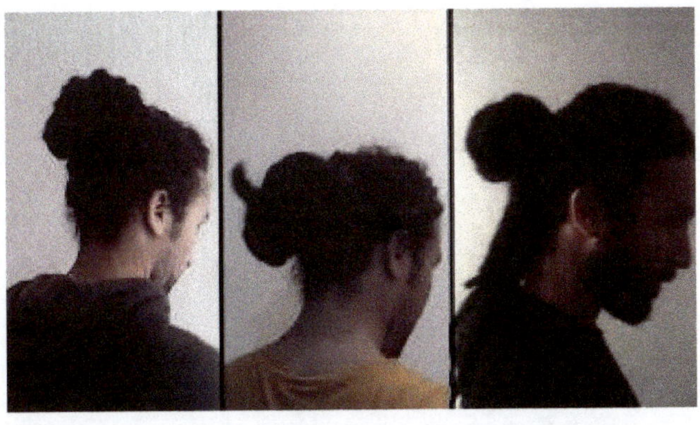

OTHER HAIR STYLES

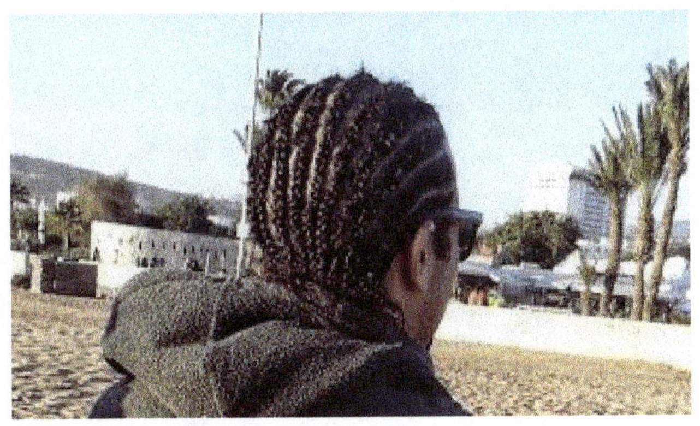

On my dreadlock journey, waiting for my hair to get long enough and to start dreading, I did try few hairstyles, there's nothing wrong with that, I invite everyone to try different things to see what suits them most, life is a journey, I must say that dreadlocks is what I want and what I was going for, but I also wanted to have some kind of memories with other outlooks, I do not judge anyone who has any kind of style as I do not like to be judged. I do not believe in trends or fashion, I do not get the concept that a bunch of people will be dictating me what to wear and what kind of haircut I'm going to have in the Spring of next year or what would be the dominant color and hairstyle in upcoming summer and I have to obey like a good boy.. no way! I like doing what I want whenever I want and however I want it.. does not matter if it is "outdated" or no longer a trend, as long as I feel good about it, because that is what it's all about, feeling good, as long as I am happy with what I am wearing and the hairstyle I am having then that's what matters.

<u>AFRO</u>

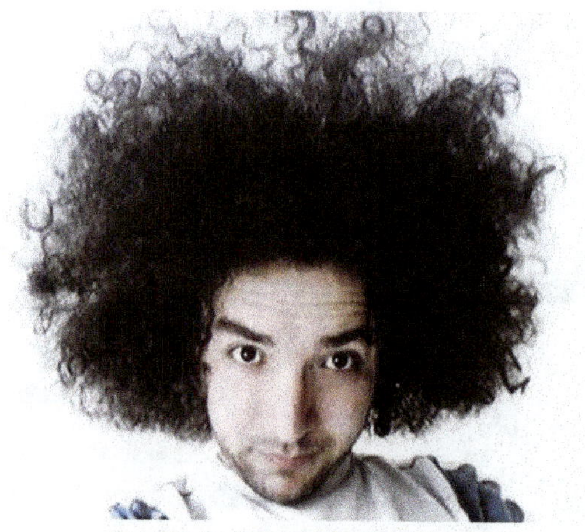

Many people like the afro look for their hair, or sometimes they want to attend an event or something and they just want to try something new, exotic and different. But their hair is straight and can't get naturally afro, there are few tutorials on YouTube that show you how to turn your straight hair into afro, for men and women, and also for short and long hair.

For my hair, it's naturally curly, so I don't have a problem to achieve the afro-ish look, using just an afro comb (or any comb that has long teeth) I could even just use my fingers, or you could use a fork.

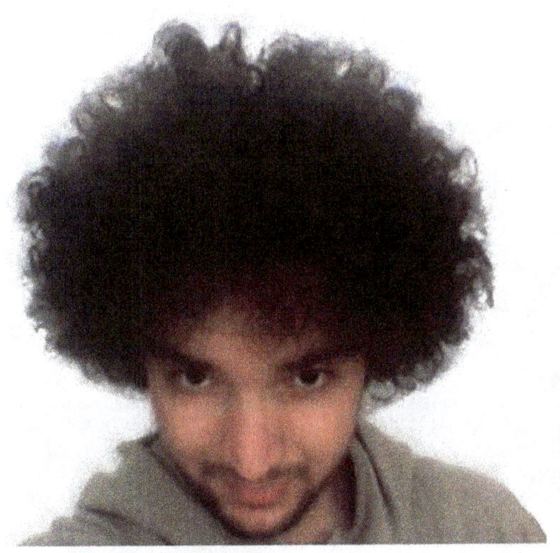

Info about Afro hair:

Afro, sometimes shortened to 'fro and also known as a "natural", is a hairstyle worn naturally by people with lengthy kinky hair texture or specifically styled in such a fashion by individuals with naturally curly or straight hair. The hairstyle is created by combing the hair away from the scalp, allowing the hair to extend out from the head in a large, rounded shape, much like a halo, cloud or ball.

In persons with naturally curly or straight hair, the hairstyle is typically created with the help of creams, gels or other solidifying liquids to hold the hair in place. Particularly popular in the African-American community of the late 1960s, the hairstyle is often shaped and maintained with the assistance of a wide-toothed comb colloquially known as an afro pick.

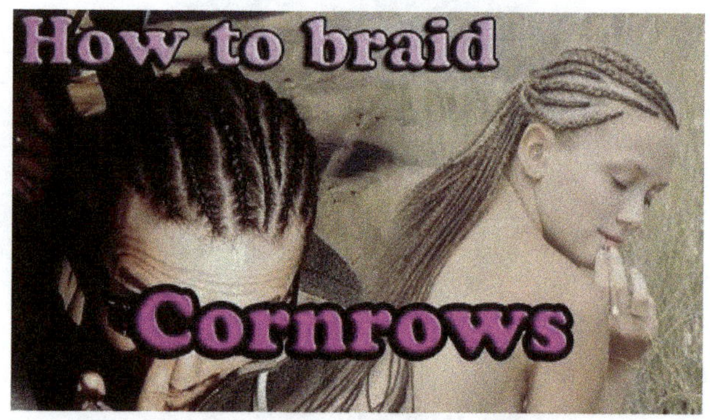

Cornrows were a phase that I have been through during my dreadlocks journey, as I said it's nice to try different exotic hairstyles sometimes.
This is not actually the first time I do this hairstyle, I have had my hair braided before twice, but I must say, the second time I have had cornrows on my hair was the best, I loved the look.

This is how to braid cornrows:
Start by sectioning the hair, choose big or small sections depending on the look you want,
Then divide the section into three small sections,
One hand holds two sections and the other hand holds the third one.
The hand that has two sections twists them to make the outer section becomes in the middle then the other hand grabs the middle section,
Then you do the same thing with the other hand.

Every time you grab the middle section grab some hair from the scalp with it, to keep the braid attached to the scalp.

You can also braid extensions with your cornrows to give your hair some extra-length.

It is better if you get human hair extensions of course, but other kinds of extensions will work fine too especially if you use them only at the back of your hair also because you will only have them on for few days.

You may also use extensions from the root of your hair if you want big and thick braids.

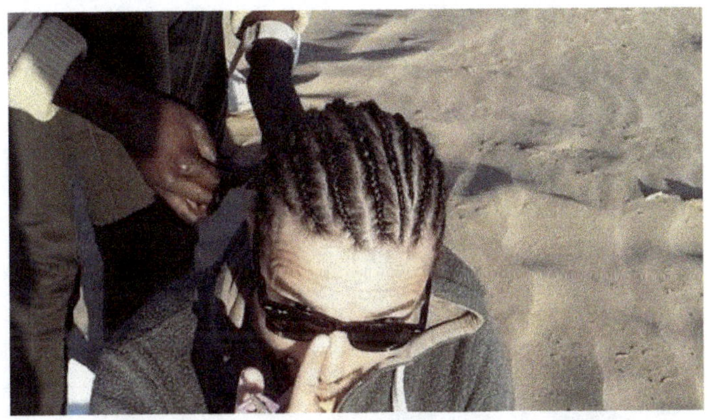

Info about Braids and Cornrows:

Cornrows, also known as braids, are a traditional African style of hair grooming where the hair is braided very close to the scalp, using an underhand, upward motion to produce a continuous, raised row. Cornrows are often formed, as the name implies, in simple, straight lines, but they can also be formed in complicated geometric or curvilinear designs. Often favored for their easy maintenance, cornrows can be left in for weeks at a time if maintained through careful washing of the hair and regular oiling of the scalp.

Cornrowed hairstyles are often adorned with beads or cowry shells, in the African and Caribbean tradition. Depending on the region of the world, cornrows are typically worn by either men, women or both. Cornrows are known as canerow in parts of the Caribbean and the United Kingdom.

MAN BUN

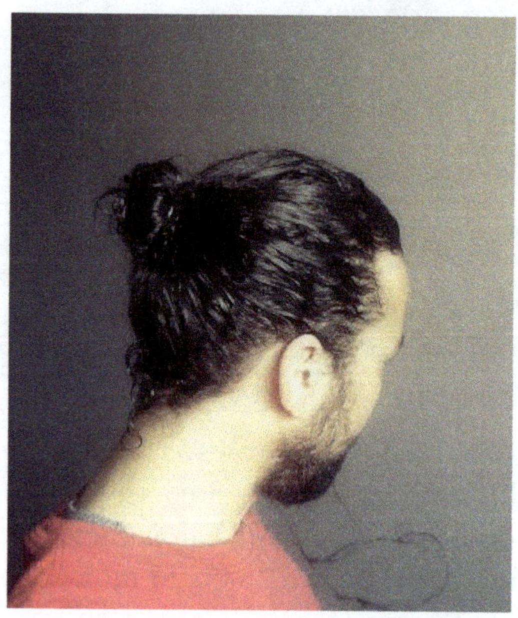

First of all, your hair must be long enough to form a bun, it does not have to be very long just long enough, you may use a natural hair cream and blow dryer.. then the rest is quiet obvious.

What's a bun?
A bun is a type of hairstyle wherein the hair is pulled back
from the face, twisted or plaited, and wrapped in a circular
coil around itself, typically on the back of the head or neck.
A bun can be secured with a barrette, bobby pins, a hair
stick, a hairnet, and/or a pencil. Buns may be tightly
gathered, or loose and more informal.
Man bun?
The term **"man bun"** is a term used to describe long-haired
men who do not wish to sport the traditional trend of short
back and sides. Men with long hair tend to use this style for
practicality and heat relief rather than a particular fashion or
trend.

But man bun is not a one specific haircut or hairstyle.. there
are many hairstyles that people call man bun, the most
popular ones are:

Full man bun: long hair on all sides, pulled back into a large
high bun.
Low man bun: Same as full man bun, but the position o the
bun is lower on the head.
Top knot: A smaller back bun using only the hair on top of
the head, side hair is shaved or just clipped.
The pineapple: Similar to the top knot but the bun is in the
center of the top hair, the pineapple bun is quite small.
The undercut: Similar to the top knot except that there's no
bun, just a smaller shoot of hair that looks like a micro
ponytail.

Samurai bun: Long hair on all sides but only the top hair is
pulled back to form a bun, the rest of the hair is left like it is.

MYTHS & FACTS ABOUT DREADLOCKS

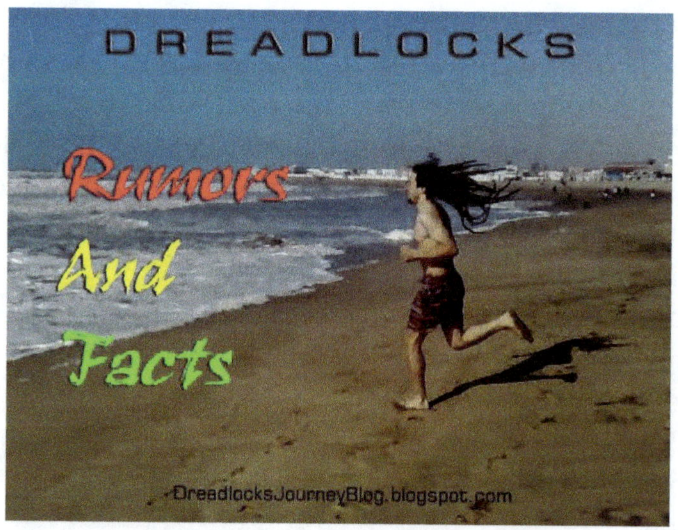

Dreadlocked hair is one of the most misunderstood hairstyles. Throughout my dreadlocks journey, I have heard many rumors and myths about dreadlocks, people seem to ignore everything.

here are the top rumors you may come across, and the facts about them:

Rumor 1

To have dreadlocks you must stop washing your hair, it needs to be dirty to lock

Fact: dirty hair is not healthy and it dreads slower, your hair must be clean to dread fast, you wash your dreadlocks just like you used to do before, except that you don't comb, and you use a residue free shampoo.

Rumor 2
Only black people can have dreadlocks, or it only suits black people.
Fact: If that was the case than people who don't have straight hair are not allowed to straighten it either, and people should never dye their hair. Dreadlocks are for everyone, all races, it sure take more time in some hair textures, but it's absolutely for everyone.

Rumor 3
Dreadlock people smoke weed or they are potheads
Fact: Not true, many people who wear dreadlocks are not rastas (even rasta people use marijuana in a controlled way) many of them don't even smoke and have a different outlook on life.

Rumor 4
You must put some product on your hair to have dreadlocks, Products you may hear that they are good for dreadlocks: Honey, Toothpaste, Glue, Chewing-gum, Mayonnaise, Candle wax, hair Gel...
Fact: Not true, do not put anything on your hair because it's unhealthy, it will become dirty and you will damage the scalp. your hair will lock itself with no help, it doesn't need any product, just patience.

But if you still want to, then use natural healthy products.

Rumor 5
Dreadlocks damage your scalp, or will make you lose hair.
Fact: Not true, if you don't use anything on your hair, and

you wash it regularly, nothing will happen to it, losing hair is related to many other factors like genetics.

Rumor 6

To remove dreadlocks you must shave your head

Fact: Not true, you can remove your dreadlocks, it's a hard process but it can still be done.

Rumor 7

The only Natural method to have dreadlocks is the neglect/freeform method

Fact: I would say it's the most natural way, but some hair textures will take a long time to lock, with a little backcombing or twisting, the process would be faster, that's all, they're still natural methods.

Rumor 8

Rubber bands will break your hair

Fact: If used in the right way, rubber bands help sectioning your hair and help tightening the roots especially on new formed dreads, and they are used only for a short period of time.

Rumor 9

Dreadlocks are for Rastas only.

Fact: Rastas did not invent dreadlocks. Cavemen used to have dreadlocks because the comb wasn't invented yet, dreadlocks are for everyone and for many reasons: fashion, spirituality, religion... whatever is good for you

Rumor 10

A funny one, after shaving your dreadlocks, your new hair will grow as dreads.

Fact: your hair just grows, your scalp doesn't even know you have dreadlocks.

BONUS

THE POTENTIAL HEALTH BENEFITS AND DRAWBACKS OF WEARING DREADLOCKS

While dreadlocks can be a beautiful and unique hairstyle, it is important to consider the potential health benefits and drawbacks before deciding to wear them.

One of the potential health benefits of dreadlocks is that they can promote hair growth. When the hair is locked, it is protected from daily manipulation such as brushing and combing, which can lead to breakage and damage. As a result, the hair is able to grow longer and stronger.

Another potential benefit of dreadlocks is that they can help to keep the scalp and hair clean. The tight, compact nature of dreadlocks can help to trap dirt and oil, making it easier to wash and clean the hair. This can lead to healthier looking hair and a cleaner scalp.

However, there are also potential drawbacks to wearing dreadlocks. One of the main concerns is the risk of scalp irritation or infection. If dreadlocks are not properly maintained and cleaned, they can become a breeding ground for bacteria and fungus. This can lead to itching, flaking, and even infection.

Another potential drawback of dreadlocks is that they can be difficult to manage and maintain. The hair must be regularly washed and re-twisted or braided to keep the dreads tight and intact. This can be time-consuming and require a significant commitment of time and effort.

It's also worth noting that some employers and workplaces may have policies or biases against dreadlocks and other natural hairstyles, which could limit professional opportunities for those who choose to wear them.

In conclusion, dreadlocks can be a beautiful and unique hairstyle, but it's important to consider the potential health benefits and drawbacks before deciding to wear them. If you decide to get dreadlocks, make sure to keep them clean, maintain them properly, and seek medical attention if you notice any signs of scalp irritation or infection. It's also important to understand the possible impact that it could have in professional and social situations.

RELATIONSHIP BETWEEN DREADLOCKS AND SPIRITUALITY OR RELIGION

Dreadlocks are particularly associated with spiritual or religious practices and beliefs of people from Africa and the Caribbean, where the hairstyle has been worn for centuries.

One of the most well-known associations between dreadlocks and spirituality is with Rastafarianism. Rastafarians are a religious movement that originated in Jamaica in the 1930s. They believe in the spiritual power of dreadlocks as a symbol of their rejection of Babylon, which they see as a symbol of oppression and materialism. Rastafarians believe that letting the hair grow naturally into dreadlocks is a way of honoring God and the natural state of their hair.

In many ancient African cultures, dreadlocks were worn by holy men and women as a symbol of spiritual attainment and devotion. In these cultures, the hairstyle was often associated with the spiritual practice of asceticism, which involves renouncing worldly desires and attachments in pursuit of spiritual enlightenment.

Some people also use dreadlocks as a spiritual practice of self-discipline and personal growth, in certain spiritual traditions like Hinduism, Jainism, Buddhism, and even in ancient Egypt, where it is believed that the pharaohs wore locks as a symbol of their divine power. Dreadlocks are seen as a sign of devotion, humility and sacrifice and a reminder to stay focused on spiritual pursuits.

Another association of dreadlocks and spirituality is that it is seen as a way of connecting to one's African heritage and

African identity, and a symbol of resistance against the forced assimilation that many communities of color have faced.

THE BUSINESS OF STARTING AND MAINTAINING DREADLOCKS AS A PROFESSION

Starting dreadlocks is a process that requires skill and patience. It involves separating the hair into sections, and then twisting or braiding the hair to create the dreadlock. This process can take several hours, depending on the length and thickness of the hair. Once the dreadlocks are started, they will need to be maintained regularly to keep them looking neat and tidy.

Maintaining dreadlocks involves a number of tasks, such as re-twisting or re-braiding the hair, cleaning and conditioning the dreadlocks, and removing any loose hair or buildup. This process can take several hours, depending on the length and thickness of the dreadlocks, and the amount of maintenance required.

The business of starting and maintaining dreadlocks as a profession, is a growing and profitable one. Many hairstylists, barbers, and salon owners have started to offer dreadlock services, as more and more people are looking to wear this unique hairstyle. There are also many independent dreadlock stylists who work as freelancers or run their own business.

There are different ways to start a business as a dreadlock stylist, some people may choose to learn the skills and techniques by themselves and start their own business, others may choose to get certifications or trainings to improve their skills and knowledge. The price for starting and maintaining dreadlocks can vary depending on the stylist's level of expertise, location, and the type of dreadlock service.

It's important to note that starting and maintaining dreadlocks as a profession, requires knowledge of hair care and proper techniques to avoid damage to the hair. It's also important to understand the cultural significance of dreadlocks and to be respectful of the client's heritage and reasons for wanting dreadlocks.

BOB MARLEY

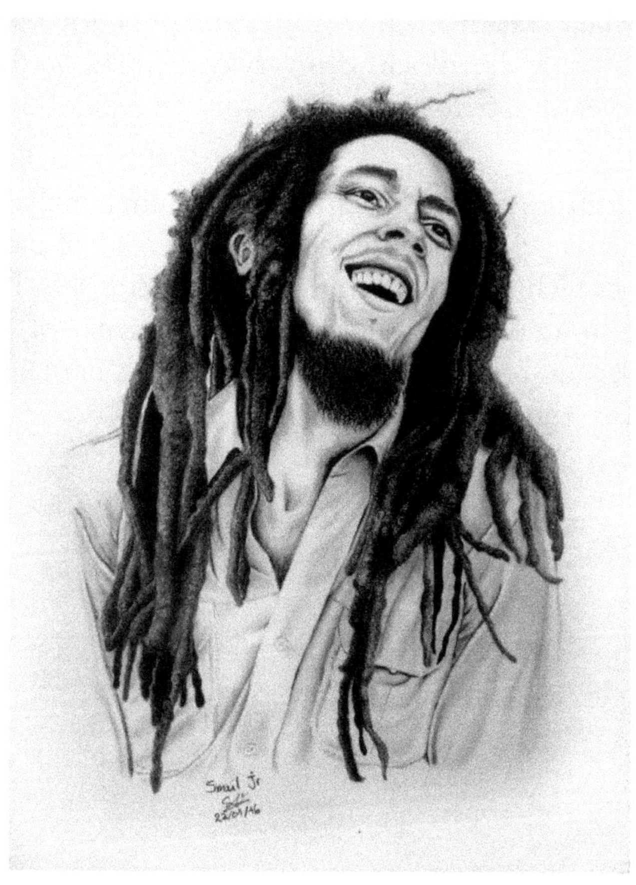

Bob Marley was the first person who inspired me to start my dreadlocks journey. It all started when I was 7-8 years old when my older brother used to listen to him and had a big poster in his room.

The look of his dreadlocks was fascinating to me, I did not know at the time what was it or what is it called or how it is done, I just wanted the same look. and also I must say from that point I really started being a fan of reggae music.

I wanted to draw Bob Marley for so long but his natty dreads made me keep delaying it, because I knew it will take too long to draw, there are too many details. But this time I made up my mind, I had to do it.

Used about four pencils, a lighter pencil, a darker one, a very dark pencil and a very sharp one for the small details. an eraser of course and a paper blending stick.

The drawing took me about 4 days, yes 4 days and a lot of energy and focus, that's because I wanted it to be one of my best Artworks and Also like I said, it has so many details.

LINKS

My YouTube channel:
www.youtube.com/DreadlocksJourney

My Instagram community page:
www.instagram.com/Dreadlocksbeauty

My dreadlocks Blog:
DreadlocksJourneyBlog.blogspot.com

My facebook community page:
www.facebook.com/TheBeautyOfDreadlocks

My creations website (drawings, short movies, music...):
www.Smail-jr.com

Peace and Love